I0123217

MORE THAN JUST A

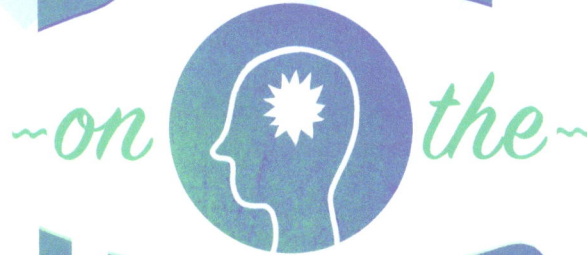

BUMP ~on~ the ~ HEAD

This book is to help you understand about a mild traumatic brain injury (TBI)*. A mild TBI is real, even if you can't see it. We hope this book will help you to understand why you feel the way you do. If you have any questions as you read through it, write them down on the inside back cover so you don't forget them. Ask your doctor at your next visit.

Contents

This book is only to help you learn. It should not be used to replace any of your doctor's advice or treatment.

* You may also hear in referred to as a mild brain injury.

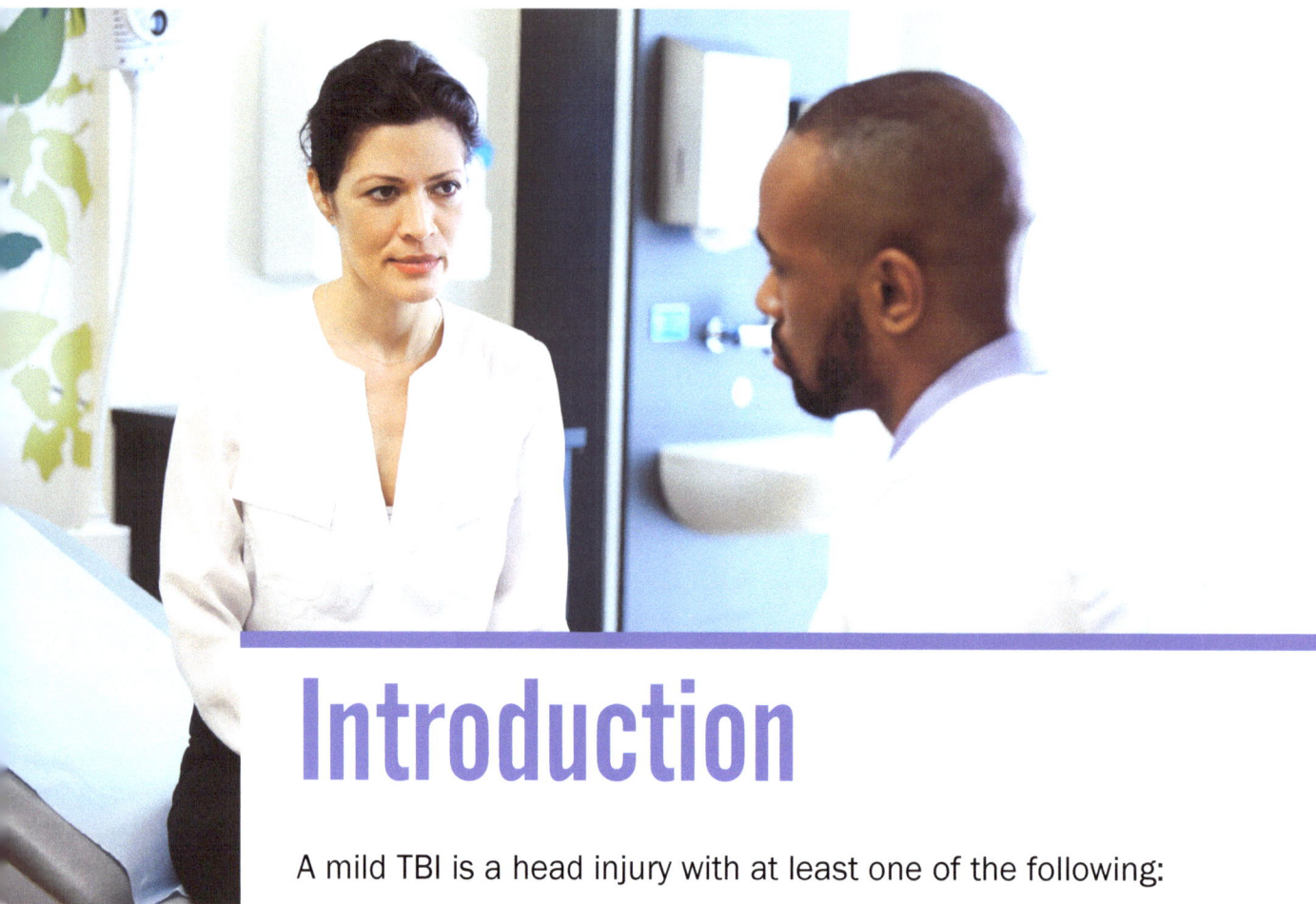

Introduction

A mild TBI is a head injury with at least one of the following:

- any change in mental status at the time of the accident

- any memory loss of what happened, before or after the accident, that does not last longer than 24 hours

- a loss of consciousness for less than 30 minutes and a GCS (Glasgow Coma Scale) score of 13–15 after you wake up

The GCS score is a way to rate a person's level of response after a head injury. It is part of the doctor's exam. It looks at responses in:

- eye movement– example: being able to open your eyes when asked

- verbal skills–example: can you carry on a clear conversation

- motor skills–example: being able to touch your nose when asked

The "unseen" injury

Thousands of people suffer brain injuries each year. Many of these injuries are severe. But some are mild traumatic brain injuries (mild TBIs).

Mild TBI is sometimes called the "unseen injury."   That's because after hitting your head, you may look and feel as if nothing is wrong. Tests may show no problems. A doctor might even say you're OK and send you home. You may not even go to a doctor and forget the injury ever happened.

But your brain may have been harmed. Without treatment, what seems like a minor injury can become a major problem.

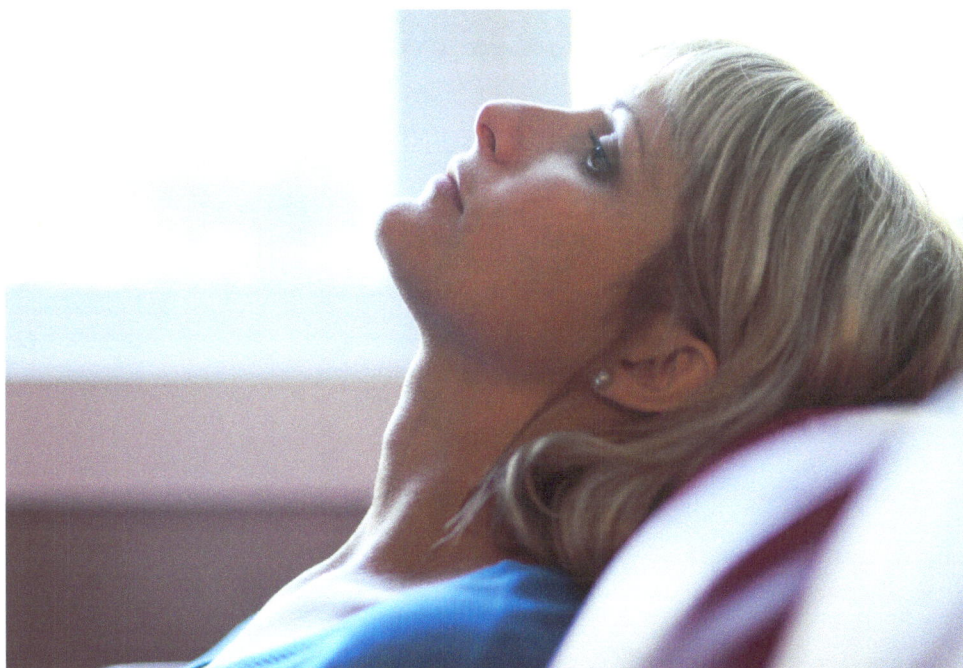

Does this sound like you?

Alice was in a car accident. She hit her head and was knocked out for a few minutes. When she woke up, her head hurt, but she didn't go to the hospital. She thought she'd feel better in a few days. But she didn't. Soon Alice didn't feel like going out with her friends anymore. She couldn't cope at work and forgot where she put things. And she didn't know what was wrong.

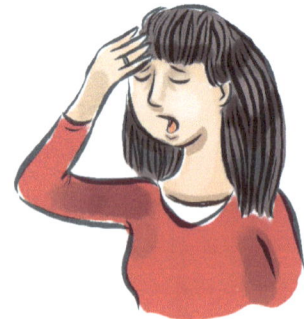

Or this?

David fell off a ladder at work and was taken to the hospital. The doctors said he'd be OK, but he had awful headaches. He couldn't control his anger or remember simple things. He couldn't smell or taste things anymore. And he felt like he was the only person in the world like this.

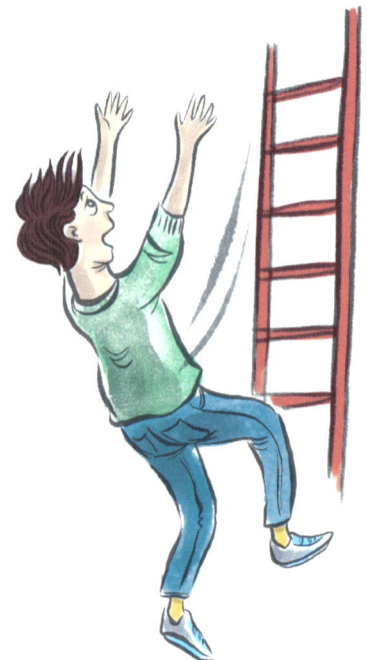

Do either of these stories sound like yours? If so, you might have a mild TBI.

What happened in my head?

A mild TBI means the brain's functions are upset by some kind of trauma—like a fall, sports injury or car accident. This is called a concussion. With a concussion, nerve fibers are stretched and torn in the brain.

Your head may not even be hit by anything. If your head is jolted, your brain may strike the inside of your skull and be hurt (as in whiplash). When your brain is bruised, it's called a contusion.

In most cases, the brain can heal itself. Your doctor may tell you to slow down and relax for a while. But if you have a sudden onset of (or drastic change in) any symptoms listed on page 6, you need to get medical help. Ask your doctor to explain any questions you may have.

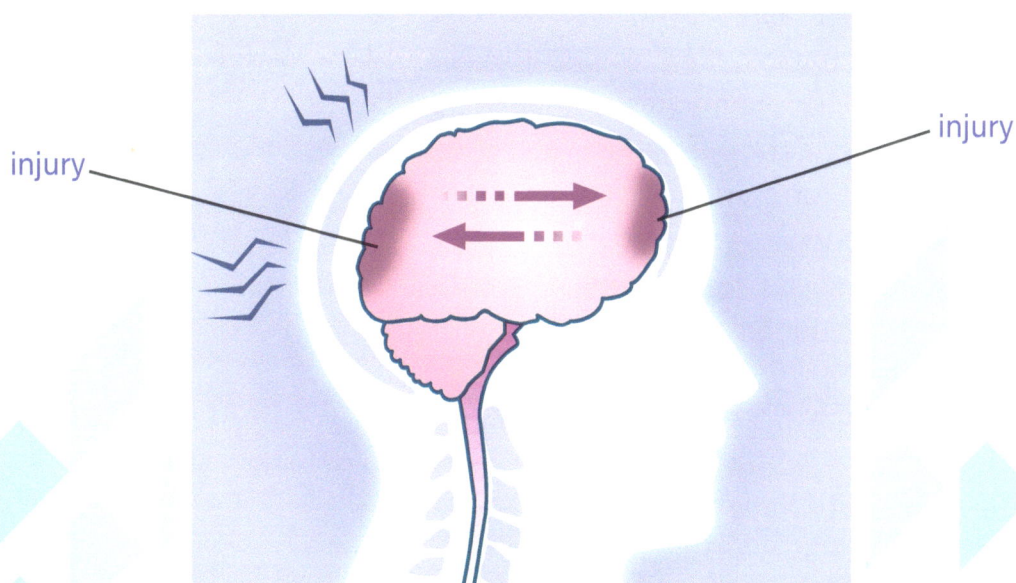

injury

injury

Signs of a mild TBI

After any head injury, watch closely for any of these signs:

- headaches, sensitivity to light and sound
- changes in speech
- differences in reaction time
- changes in judgment and trouble paying atention
- memory problems
- personality changes and bursts of emotion
- mild seizures
- loss of balance

Vomiting, trouble sleeping and nightmares are also common signs.

Oh, this headache!

You may have headaches after your injury. These are called *post-concussive headaches*. They can cause constant, mild or severe pain. Sometimes post-concussive headaches go away after a few weeks, but sometimes they don't. A headache problem may be long-term.

Two types of headaches may result from a head injury. These are vascular and tension headaches.

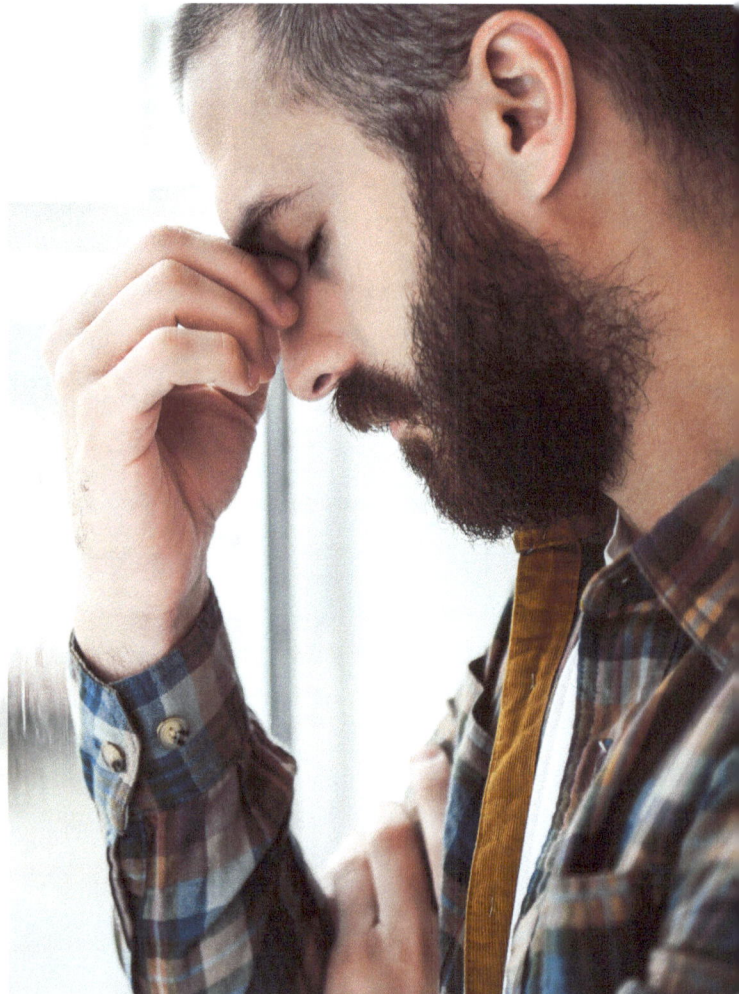

Vascular headaches

These are sometimes called migraine headaches. They result from problems with the blood vessels around your brain.

If you have a migraine headache, you may feel a hard, throbbing pain on one or both sides of your head. You may feel dizzy or sick to your stomach. **Bright lights** and **loud noises** can make your head feel worse. Migraines can pass quickly or last for many hours. They are more common in women than men.

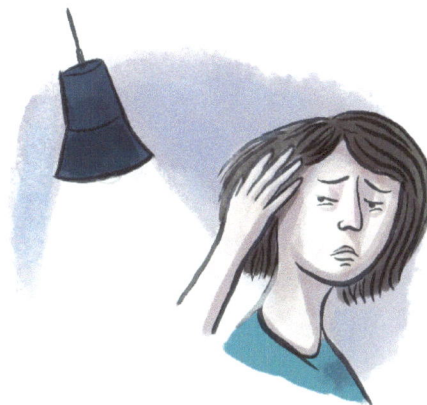

Tension headaches

These often attack when you are under stress or the muscles in your neck, shoulders or jaw are tight. The pain moves to your head and feels like a dull, steady ache.

Tension headaches can last for a long time, but they don't have to. To get rid of one, you must relax. Massage your sore spots, and put a warm towel or pad on your head and neck.

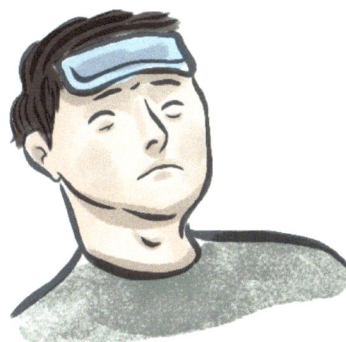

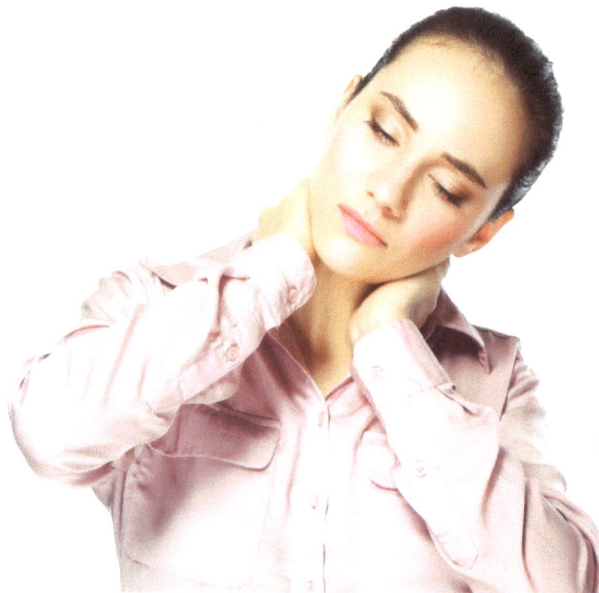

neck stretching

To manage headache pain:

- Learn what happened before the pain started, and avoid it in the future.

- Pace yourself. Work for an hour and rest for 15 minutes. Or work for 15 minutes and take a 5 minute break.

- Lie down in a dark, quiet room. Close your eyes and relax. Try to see yourself in a peaceful, relaxed place.

- Avoid loud noises.

- Stretch and/or massage the muscles in your head and neck.

- Don't let others keep you from treating your pain. They may not see your pain, but it's real.

- Admit that your headache pain might be lasting. Do your best to accept this and get along with your life.

NOTE: Read the labels on medicines like aspirin and ibuprofen before you use them. Take the right number of pills. If a medicine doesn't work, **don't take larger doses.** Call your doctor and ask for help.

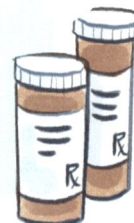

I know what to say, but . . .

Changes in speech are often a sign of a mild TBI. When your brain is hurt, it doesn't work as fast or as well. You might make mistakes, so be patient with yourself.

- **Trouble finding the right word**
  You know the word you want to use, but can't find it. Or you use the wrong words without knowing it. You might say "hotel" for hospital or "sick truck" for ambulance.

- **Trouble telling the story**
  You have a hard time telling a story that makes sense. You skip over the start, mix up the details or forget the ending. Or you repeat stories you've already told.

- **Trouble reading**
  You can't read as fast as you could before your injury. Letters look strange, and it takes you longer to know what words mean.

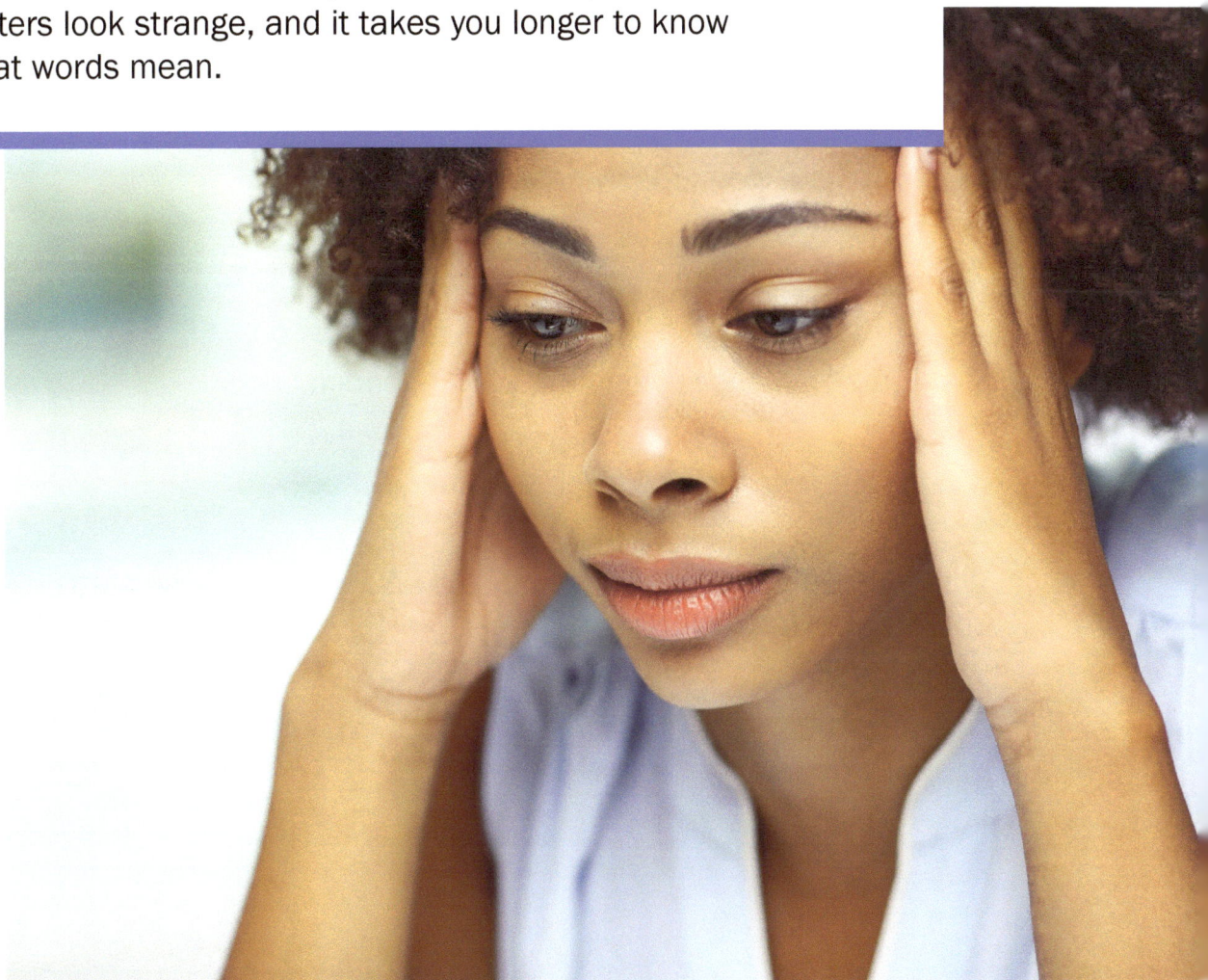

I can't get started...
I can't finish anything

Judgement is often affected by a mild TBI. Without a TBI, you would:

1. see a problem

2. think of ways to solve it

3. choose the best way

4. make a plan for solving it

5. start the plan

6. make changes along the way, if needed

7. rate your success when you finish

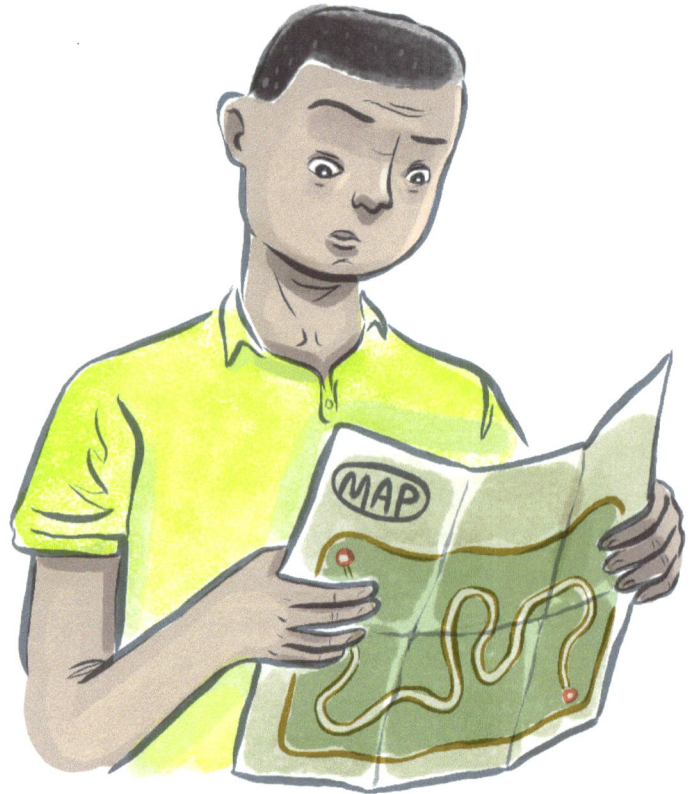

With a mild TBI, you may have trouble with some of these steps. You may not be able to start or finish anything. You may get stuck and keep doing the same step over and over. And you may not even see that you're having trouble.

These tips may help you get things done:

- Wake up and start your day at the same time each day.

- Set small goals that are easy to reach.

- Break tasks into smaller ones until you have a plan you can complete. Write your plan on paper or record in your phone or tablet.

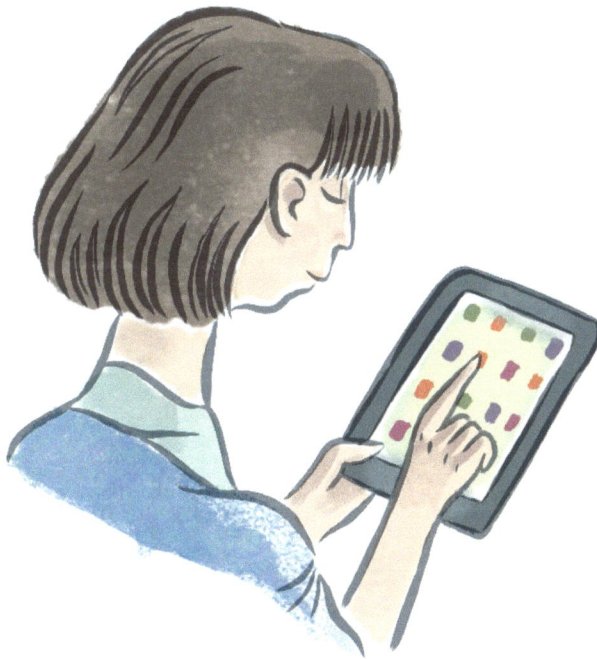

- Ask for feedback from a loved one about how you are doing.

- Think things through before you take action.

- Take a break or a nap when you are tired. You will do better when you can think more clearly.

Were you talking to me?

One sign of a mild TBI is **trouble paying attention.** You might not be able to keep your mind on anything. You may jump from one thought to another or start something in the middle of something else.

Here are 3 tips that can help:

- **Do one thing at a time.** Your brain can't juggle like it used to.

- **Pace yourself.** Slow down. Don't try to force your brain to work faster than it can.

- **Stay in quiet places.** Lights, motion and loud noises can distract you and make you nervous and grouchy.

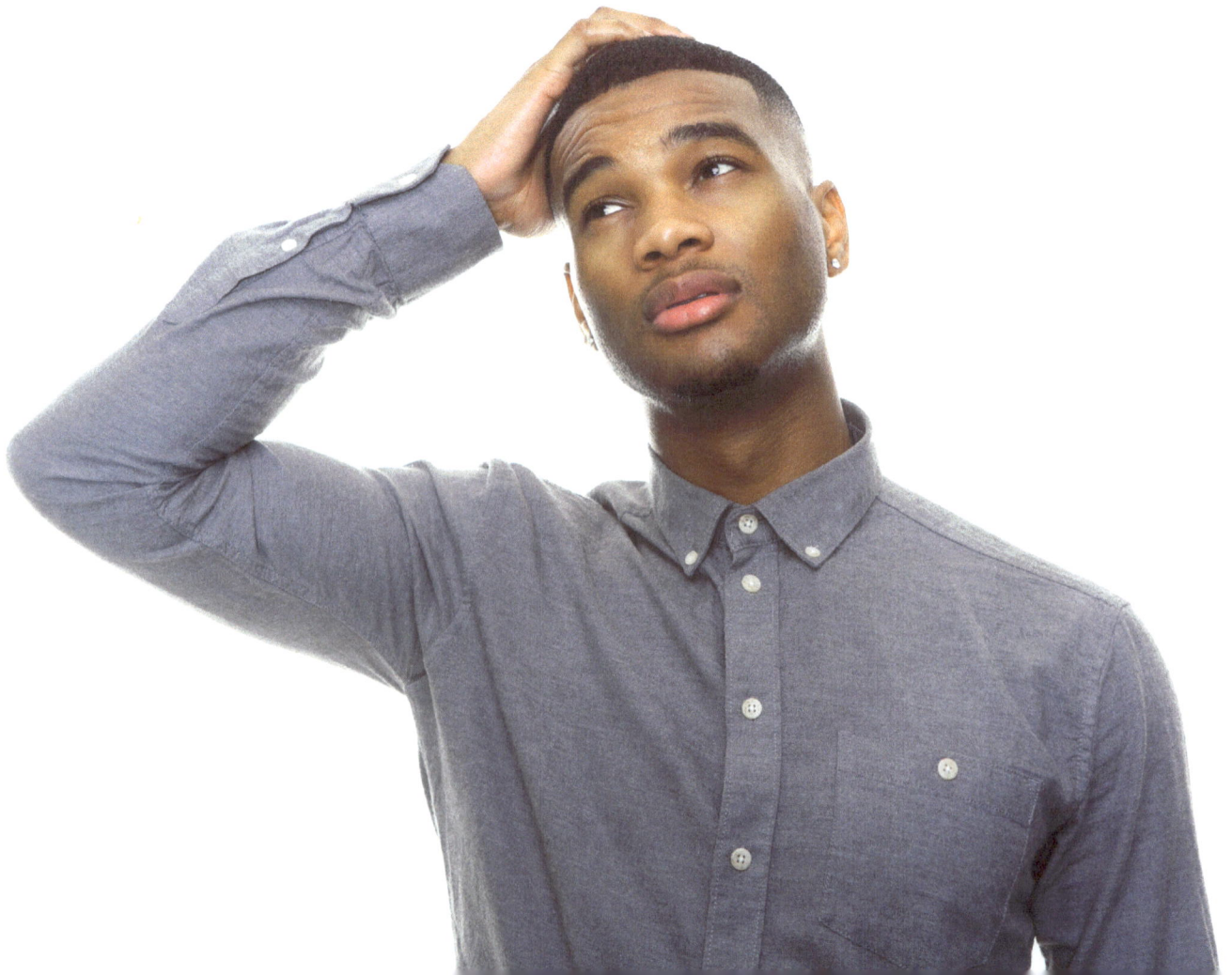

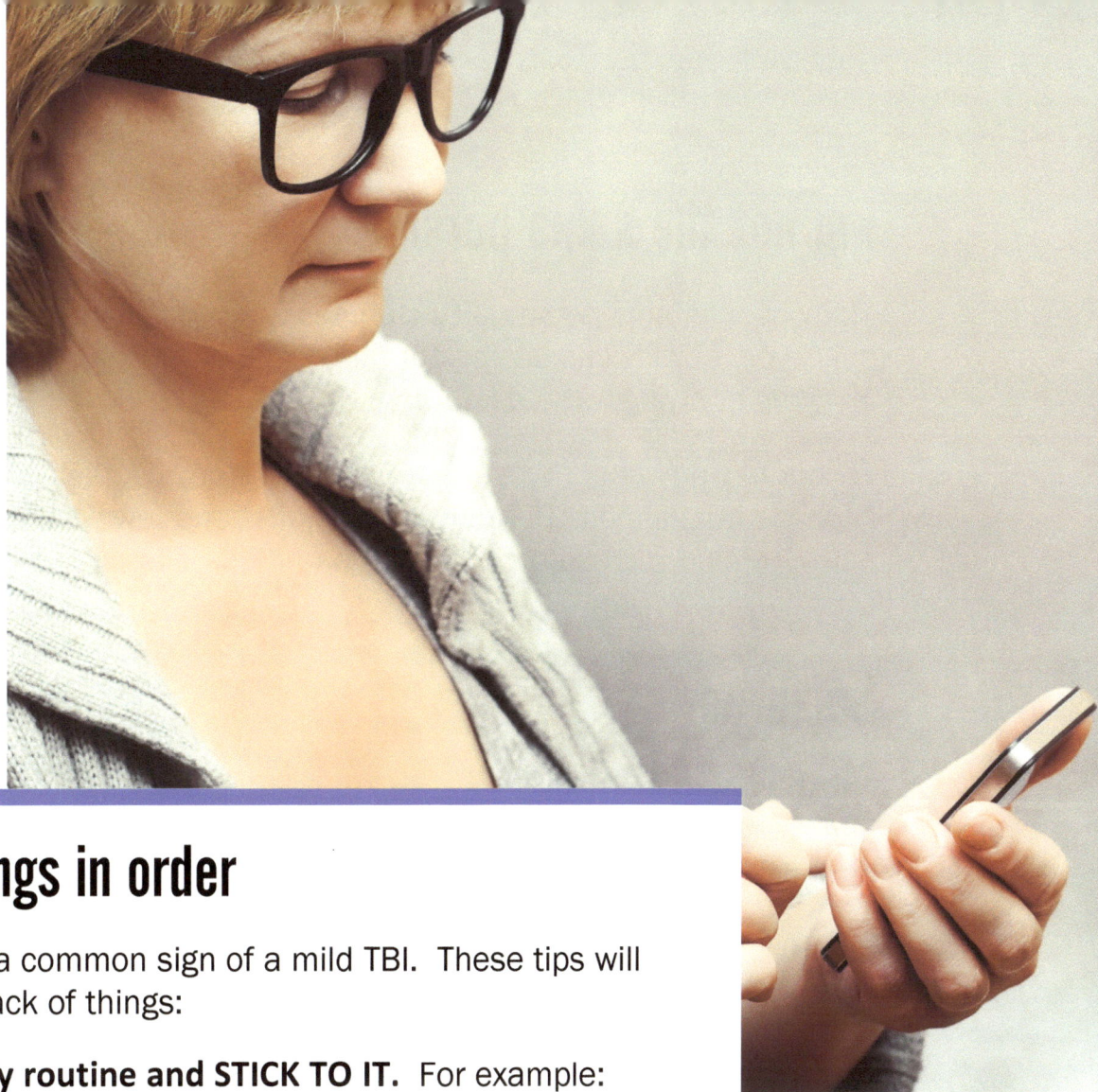

Keeping things in order

Memory loss is a common sign of a mild TBI. These tips will help you keep track of things:

- **Set up a daily routine and STICK TO IT.** For example: wake up, go to the bathroom, brush your teeth, shower, get dressed and have breakfast—in the same order every day. Plan your whole day or just the part that is tough for you.

- **Stay focused.** Don't let anyone stop or distract you from your routine. Tell them you need to finish what you are doing.

- **Keep important things in the same place.** It's hard to keep track of everything—even when your brain is fine. Try to group as many things into one place as you can. For example, keep all the things you need when you leave your house (keys, wallet, sunglasses) next to the door.

- **Keep notes or a calendar on your phone.** Write down your routines for home, work or school. Write out a "to do" list for each day. Also write down any major decisions you make. Review your schedule often each day.

I'm not the same person

Many people have **personality changes** after a brain injury. You may get angry very quickly and scare your family and friends. Or you may start laughing or crying without knowing why.

Try not to worry about these new feelings. Many people with personality changes from a mild TBI return to normal after a few weeks. If you get angry, remind yourself of your injury and try to relax.

Seizures

Seizures can be a result of a mild TBI. During a seizure, you may stare off into space and feel confused. One side of your body, or your whole body, may start shaking.

Pay attention to how you feel. Your body may send signals when a seizure is about to happen. Some signals are:

- seeing a glow (aura) around objects

- your body becoming stiff and tense

- a tingling feeling on your skin

- smelling things others don't smell

You may have a seizure during the night and wake up very sore or out of your bed. If you think you may have had a seizure, go to the emergency room right away.

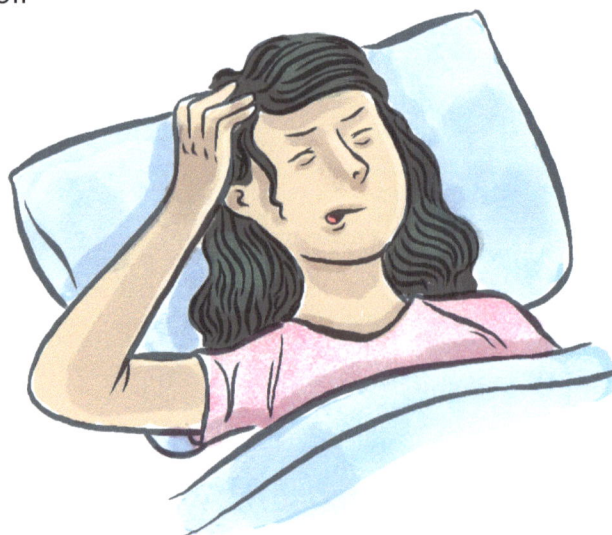

Loss of balance

A mild TBI can also cause **inner ear** (vestibular) **problems.** The inner ear connections to the brain may be harmed during a brain injury.

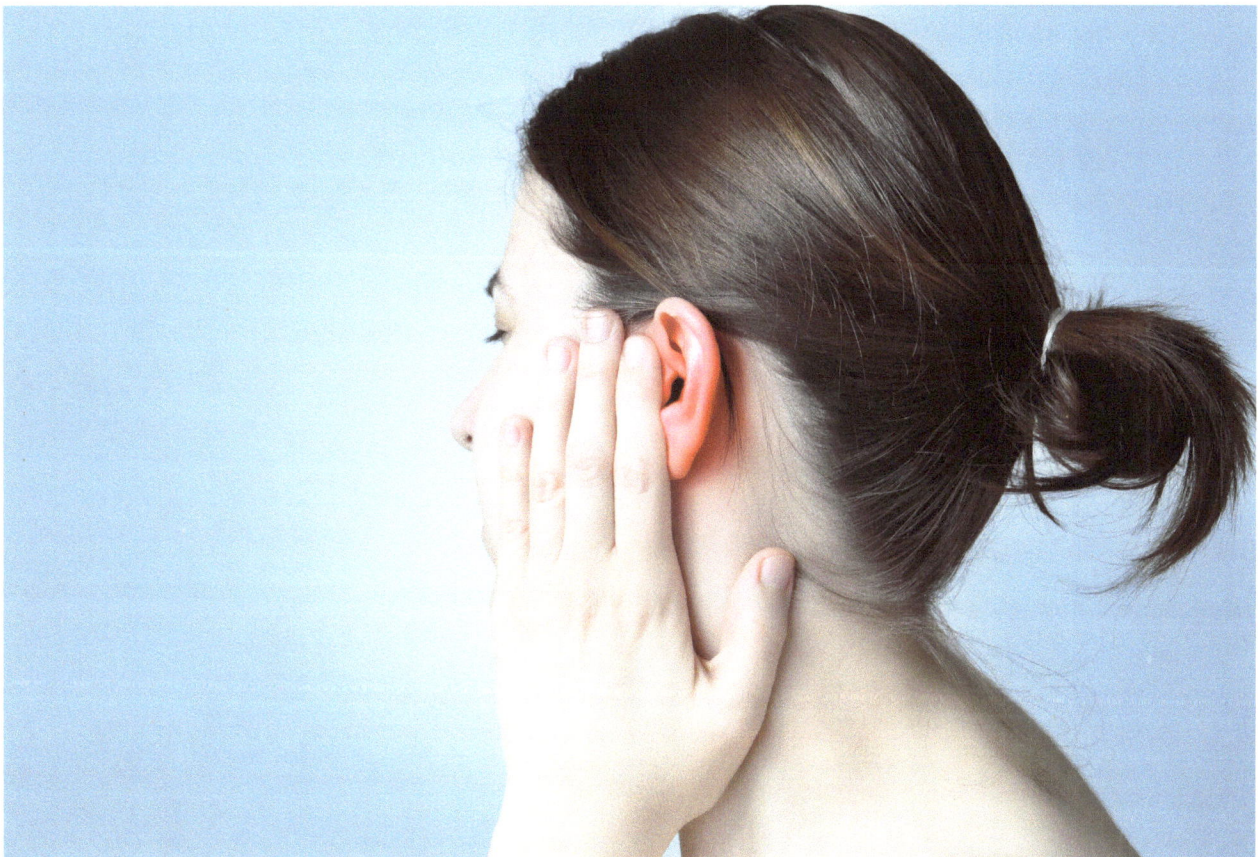

Inner ear problems may cause:

- loss of balance
- ringing in the ears
- hearing loss
- blurred vision
- dizziness, nausea
- headaches

If you have any of these problems, talk with your doctor. You may need to see an ear, nose and throat doctor. Or you may be sent to a physical therapist for special treatment.

Does my TBI affect my family?

Your family members may change the way they act around you. They may not understand your injury because you look fine. Or they may try to do everything for you.

You were the one injured, but your family has suffered too. Just like you, they may feel a sense of loss. Be aware of their feelings.

Talk with your loved ones about changes in you and in them. Share this book with them to help them understand. Communication makes things easier for everyone.

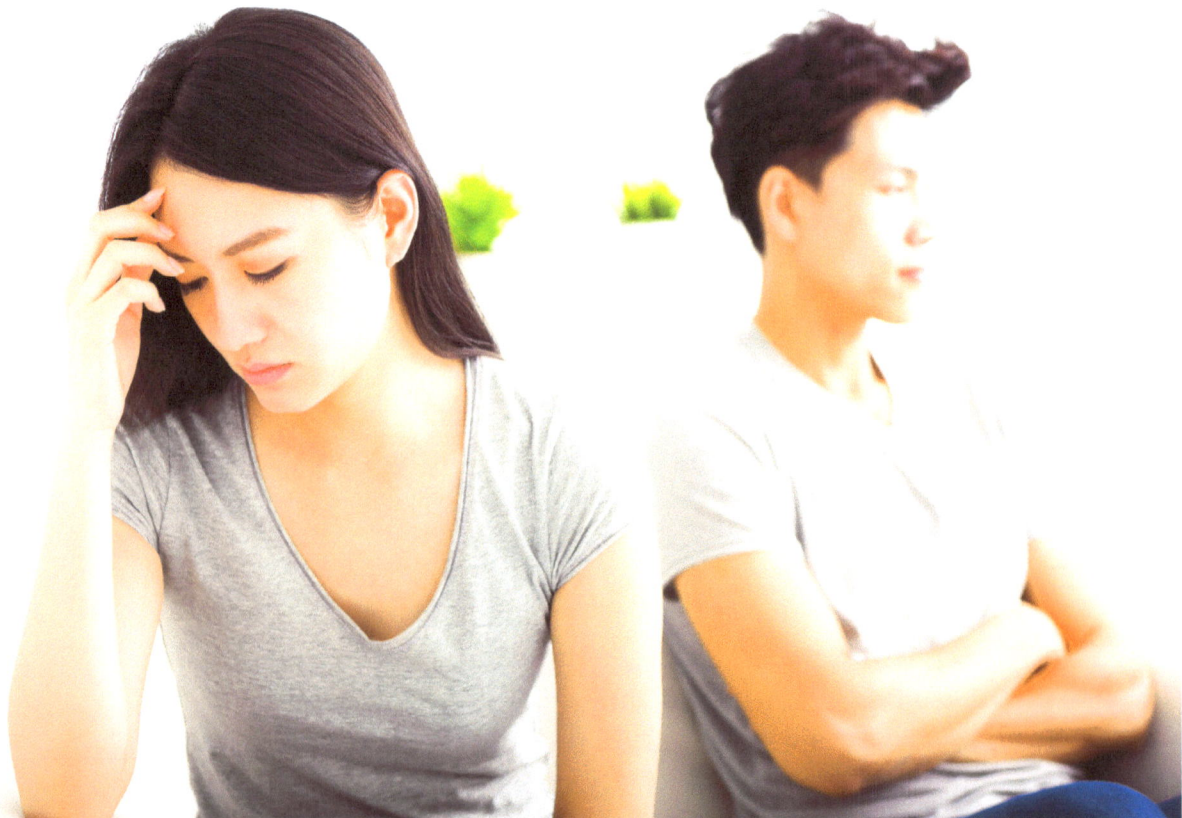

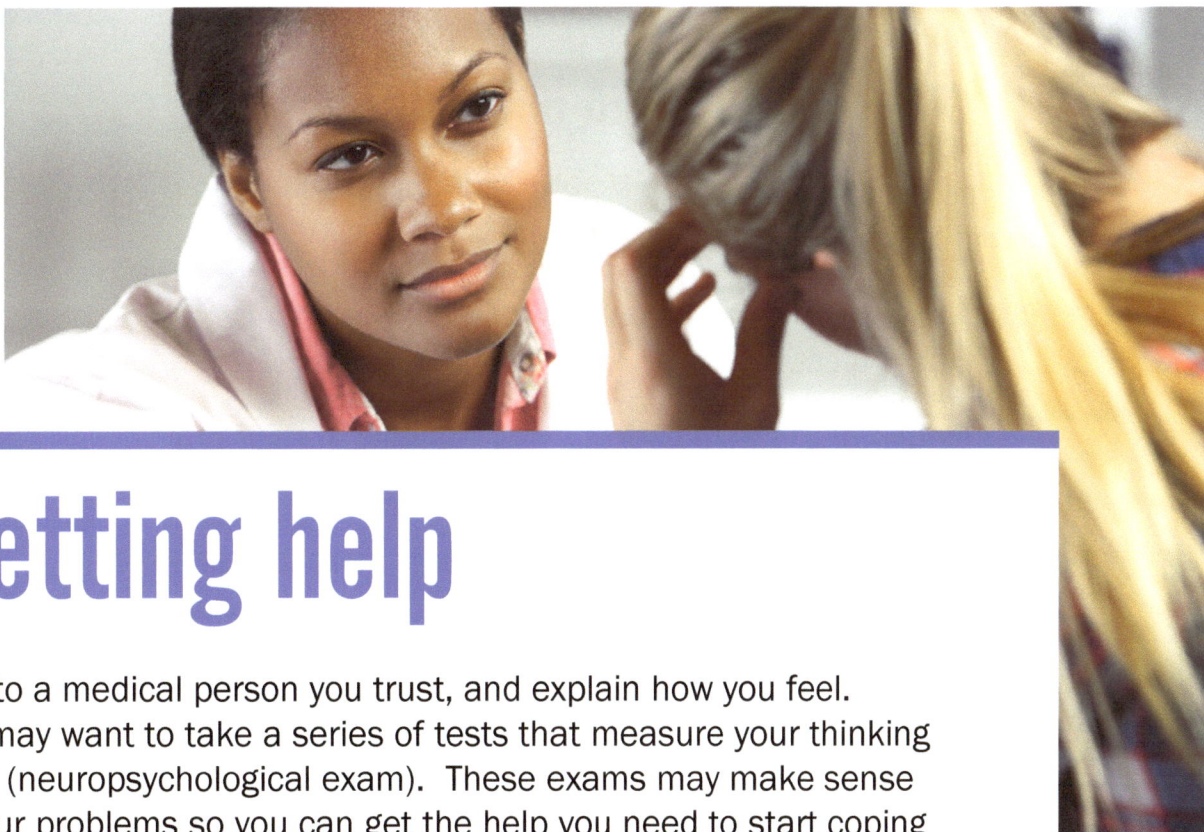

Getting help

Talk to a medical person you trust, and explain how you feel. You may want to take a series of tests that measure your thinking skills (neuropsychological exam). These exams may make sense of your problems so you can get the help you need to start coping with the changes.

Contact the **Brain Injury Association** (biausa.org). They can give you information for local support groups and things to read about brain injuries.

Therapy

You may need therapy to help you learn to cope. There are many types of therapy. It could mean seeing one or more of these:

- neuropsychologist

- speech/language pathologist

- cognitive rehabilitation therapist

- physical therapist

- occupational therapist

- rehabilitation counselor

Talk to your doctor about the sort of problems you are having so you can get the right kind of help.

Doctors are there to help you

Some doctors are trained to understand and treat problems caused by mild brain damage.

- **Neuropsychologists** study how the brain affects the way you act.

- **Neurologists** help people with problems in their brains and nervous system.

- **Physiatrists** help injured people regain strength and control over their bodies.

Keep these tips in mind:

- Ask lots of questions—even if you think they sound silly. Write down questions before you go. Then, write down answers during your doctor visit.

- Stay away from doctors who say there is nothing wrong with you. Find a doctor who explains things to you in words you understand.

- You have **real** symptoms of a **real** injury.

- Don't stop asking questions until you feel you are satisfied with the answers.

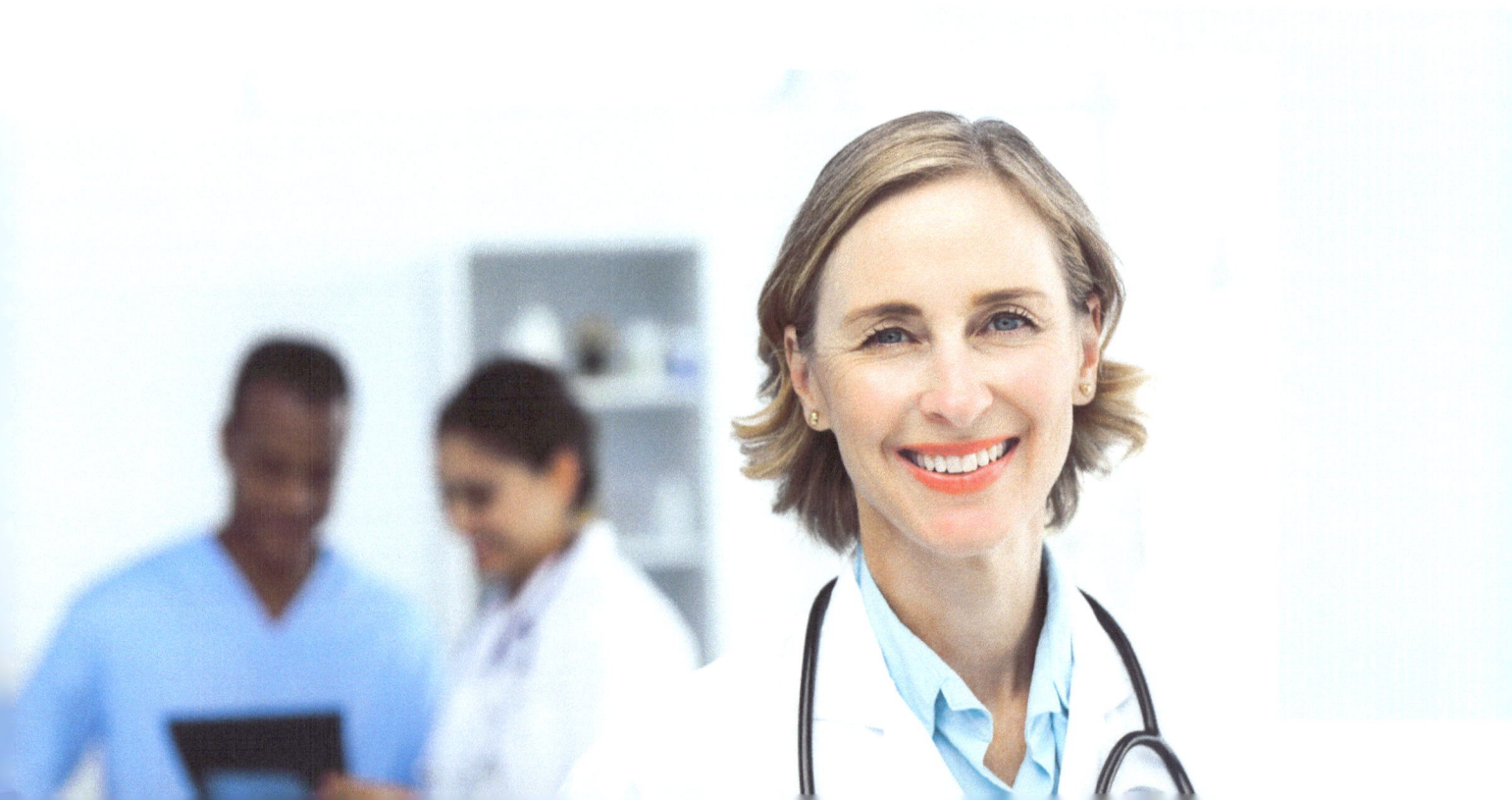

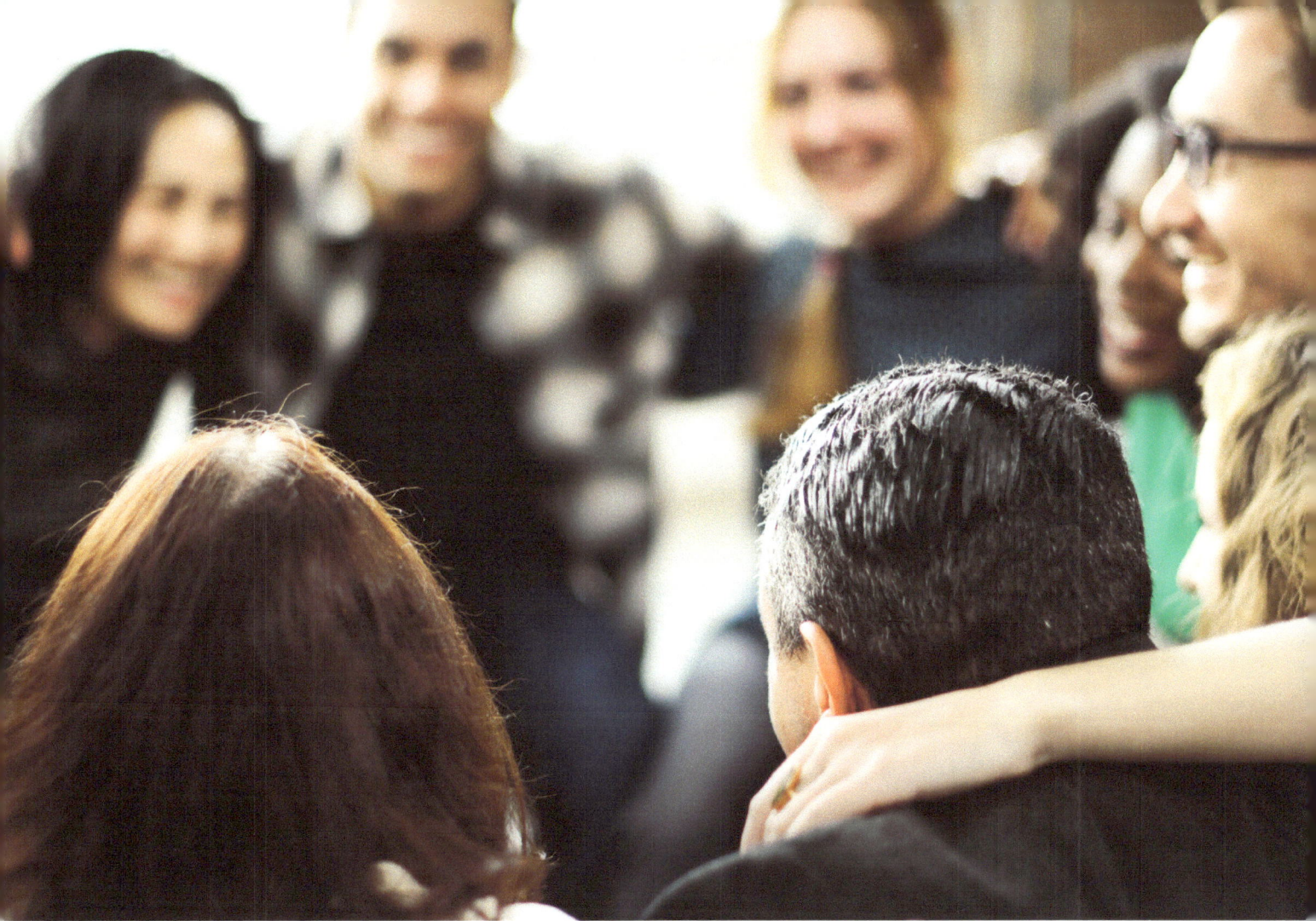

You need support

After your injury, you need the love and support of family and friends to get better. You may want to join a support group of people with injuries like yours.

Invite your family and friends to join your support group. They need to learn about mild TBI to help youfind ways to take control of your life.

Many people with mild TBIs say that their injuries have slowed them down and helped them notice the things in life that really matter. You may find that you are better able to enjoy the simple things and value the people who care about you even more.

Here are some things to keep in mind about support:

- Choose trusted friends or family members as support people. You need people who will help look out for you. This is most true right after your injury. Since you rely on them to help you recover, they need to learn about mild TBI.

- You will need more than one support person. Pick one for home, one for work or school and one for therapy.

- Trust your support people. Talk to them before you do anything important. They can give you feedback and new ideas to help you make decisions. Think about each person's opinion before you act.

- Do as much as you can for yourself. It's easy to lean on your support people too much. Don't let others do everything for you. As you improve, you will need your support people less and less.

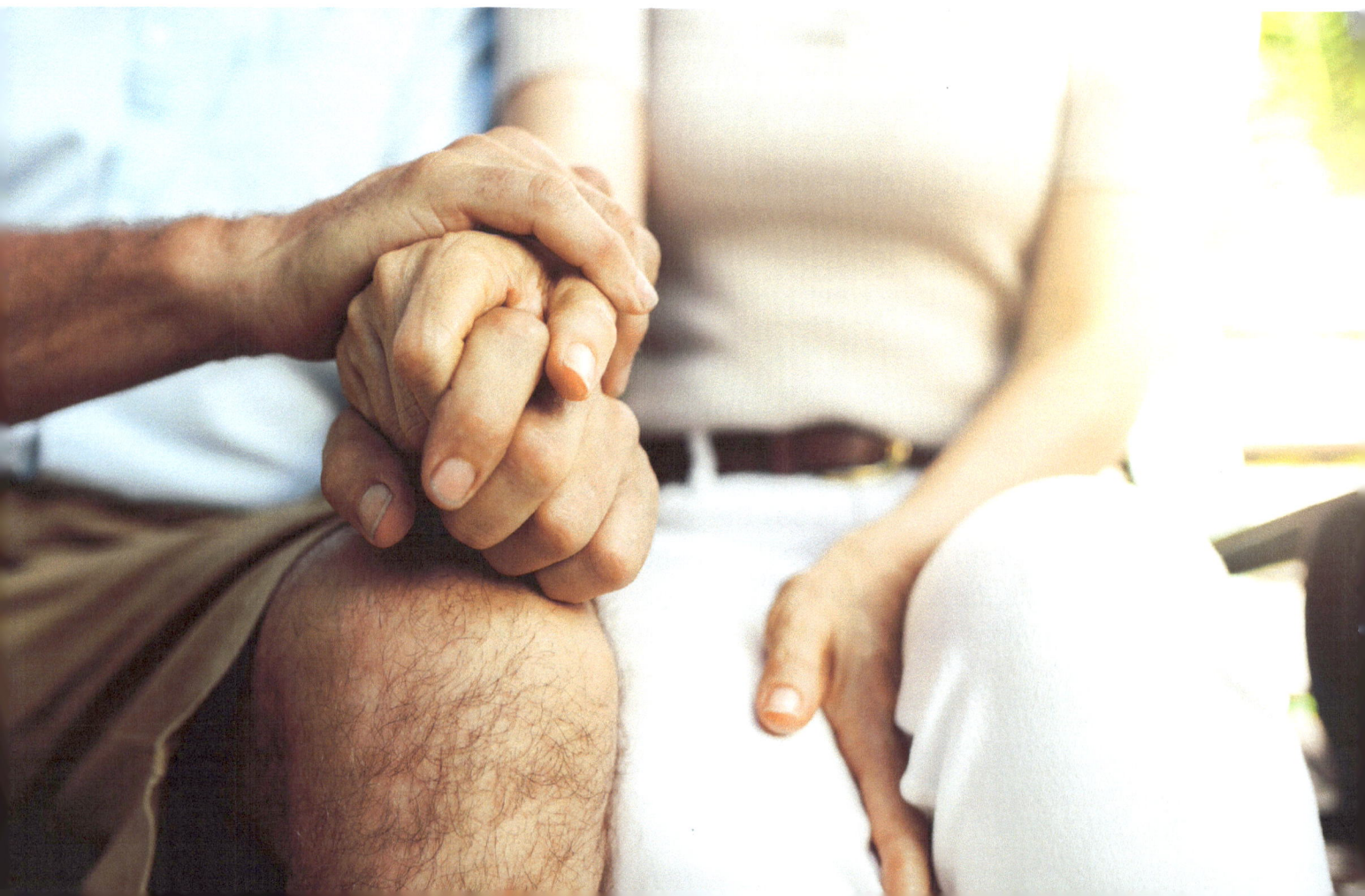

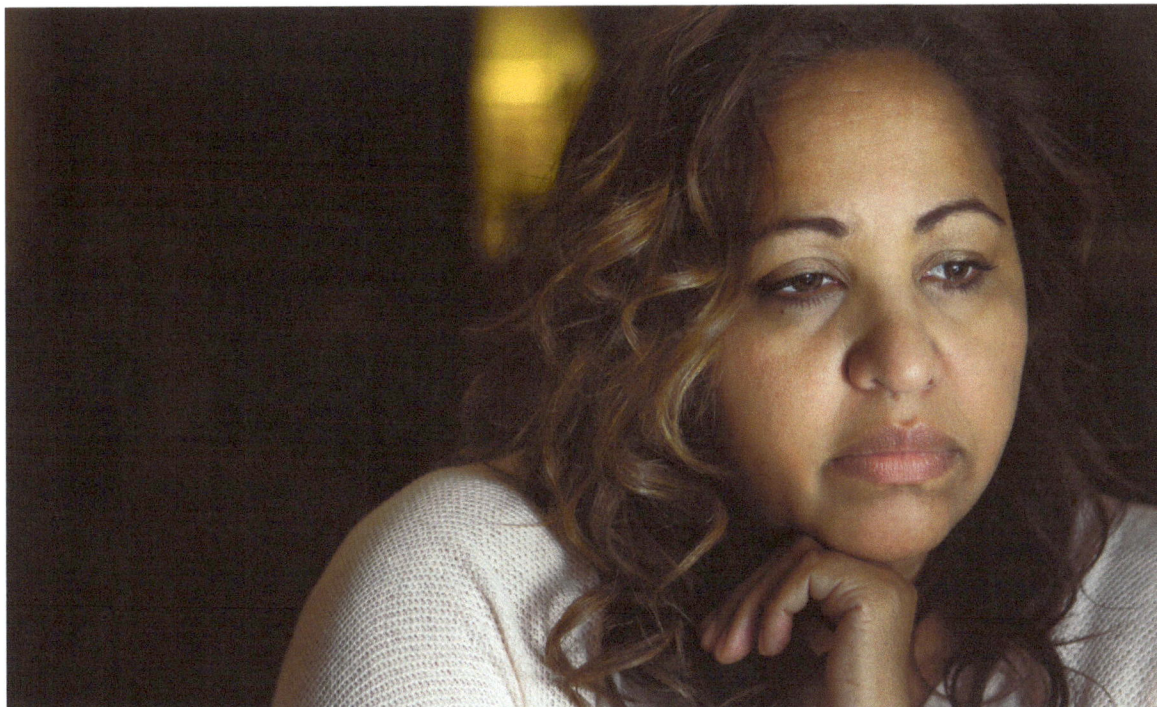

Depression

Because no one can see your mild TBI, everyone expects you to act as you did before your injury. This is the time to call on your support people. Talk to them about how you feel. Just talking about it may help you feel better.

Your depression may be a medical problem. Your injury may have hurt the part of your brain that controls your moods. You may feel like a piece of you is missing. Don't wait to get help. The right medicines and therapy will help you.

Should I tell?

Whether or not you tell people that you have a brain injury is up to you. Before you decide, talk with your support people and get their advice. You may want to tell some people and not others.

It may be best for some people to know. You may need to tell your boss or your teachers. They can change your work load. You can tell co-workers or friends if and when you feel like it.

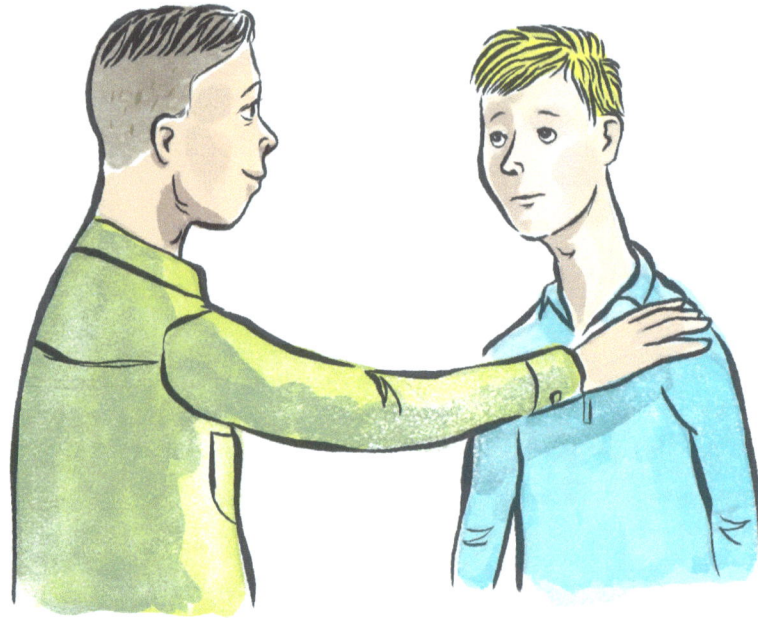

Tips for friends and family

- Accept the person with a brain injury for who he is. Don't push him to be someone else.

- Be patient. A brain takes time to heal. You don't need to see an injury for it to be there.

- Keep instructions simple and clear. Most people can understand instructions if they are given one at a time.

- Accept that what is gone may never come back.

- Let the person with a brain injury do as much as he can for himself. Treat him as you did before the injury.

- Talk **to** the person with the injury, not around him.

- Talk about the effects of the mild TBI with him. Communication will help you both.

- Learn all you can about mild TBI.

Tips for healing

Give yourself time. Your brain has been hurt, and you can't do everything you did before your injury. You may look the same, but your brain has changed.

Lighten your schedule. Get lots of rest, eat well and exercise. Make healing your top goal. Here are some tips to help you heal:

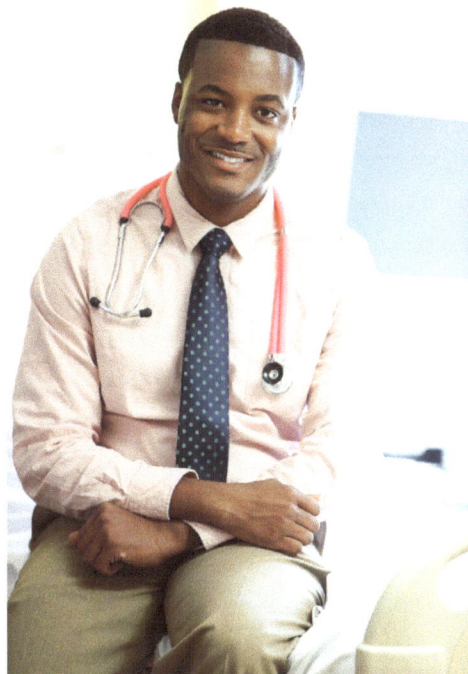

- **Don't overdo it.** Take breaks as you need to. Talk with your boss or your teachers about this.

- **Set small goals that you can reach.** Focus on one thing at a time. Break down tasks into smaller steps if you can.

- **Expect to get better slowly.**

- **Be patient** with yourself, coworkers, family and friends. If you get angry, leave the room or take a walk. Wait until you can talk calmly.

- **Do light exercise,** like walking, 3 to 5 times a week or as your doctor tells you.

- **Avoid caffeine, alcohol and other drugs.** Alcohol makes it harder for your brain to heal. It also increases the chance of seizures. Caffeine and other drugs affect your brain and change the way you think and act.

- **Don't drive.** Let someone else do the driving until your doctor says you are OK.

REMEMBER: to take the drugs your doctor prescribed for you.

The outlook is good!

Your mild TBI will most likely go away, but you must be patient. The best thing you can do to help yourself heal is learn about mild TBI. Ask your doctor all the questions you can think of. Call the Brain Injury Association (1-800-444-6443) for more information.

It may take months or years for your brain to heal. But over 85% of people who have headaches and other problems from a mild head injury have a complete recovery.

Many people with brain injuries say that healing is like being born again. They say:

"Don't let what you CANNOT do stop you from doing what you CAN."

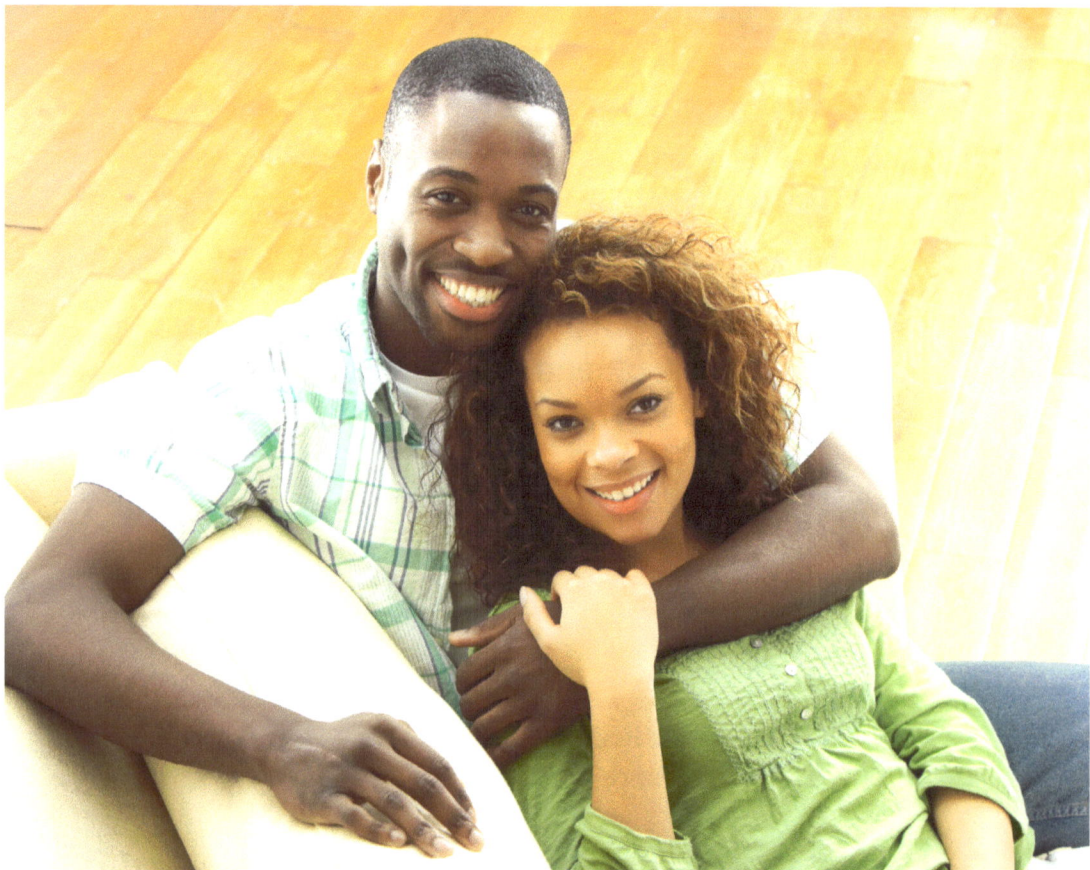

Notes and resources ✏️

Date of accident: _____

How I got hurt: _____

_____

_____

Symptoms: _____

_____

_____

Questions to ask my doctor: _____

_____

_____

_____

Additional resources

Brain Injury Association

1608 Spring Hill Road, Suite 110

Vienna, VA 22182

(800) 444-6443

www.biausa.org

Social service organizations and community groups can be valuable
resources. Members of your health care team may be able to provide
additional resources. Don't forget about support groups at your local
hospital. More importantly, take some steps toward learning what
you can do to help yourself learn more about caring for yourself or
a loved one.

® Order this book from :

PRITCHETT & HULL ASSOCIATES, INC.
3440 OAKCLIFF RD NE STE 126
ATLANTA GA 30340-3006
or call toll free: 800-241-4925

Copyright© 1996, 2005, 2013, 2017
by Pritchett & Hull Associates, Inc. All
rights reserved. No part of this book may
be photocopied, reprinted or otherwise
reproduced without written permission
from Pritchett & Hull Associates, Inc.

Published and distributed by: Pritchett & Hull
Associates, Inc. Printed in the U.S.A.

We know that you work with many health
care professionals (doctors, nurses,
physiatrists, etc.) in the management of
your mild TBI, but to keep the text simple,
we refer to your health care professionals
as "doctor" throughout the book.

www.ingramcontent.com/pod-product-compliance
Lightning Source LLC
Chambersburg PA
CBHW060855270326

41934CB00002B/153

* 9 7 8 1 9 4 3 2 3 4 1 6 5 *